THINK "NO PINK"

your bff guide to breast cancer

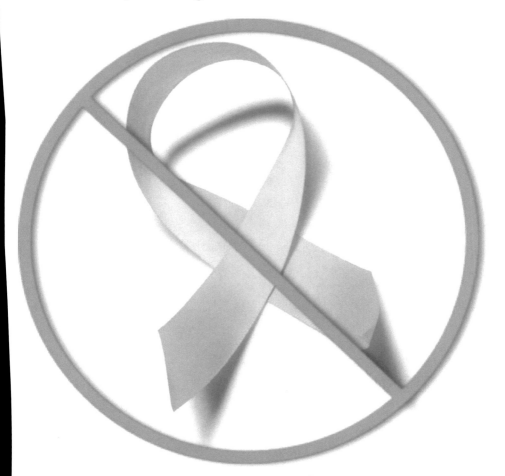

MJ JENKINS, CHC

For Reprint or Special Sales CONTACT
<u>www.ThinkNoPink.com</u>

Think "No Pink"
your BFF guide to breast cancer
©2014 MJ Jenkins

CONTENTS

Foreword

No one wants to suffer from a killer disease or health condition. It's the last thing in the world you would want to happen to you.

Today, more and more people are diagnosed with terrifying health diseases, including breast cancer. This form of health disease is common among women.

According to The American Cancer Society, one out of every eight women in America will be diagnosed with Breast Cancer.

A breast cancer diagnosis may be one of the most heart-breaking pieces of news a person can ever receive.

Women who get this diagnosis often feel depressed, and don't know what to do. This is a normal reaction, especially for a novice to breast cancer like me.

Breast cancer is not like having a fever that you can cure with just simple medication and rest. Breast cancer is a condition that requires a thorough diagnosis and professional treatment AND multiple surgeries in order to prevent it from getting worse or spreading.

This is the book that I wish had been available for me when I got my diagnosis. I've been in your shoes, I've felt what you are feeling, and I've made all the mistakes already — and thank God, I've lived to share my hard-earned wisdom and experiences, so you don't have to make the same costly errors.

Through this book, you will be able to gain better understanding of what a breast cancer really is and how will you will able to deal with it.

Facing the dreads of breast cancer is never an easy battle; so let this book guide you towards awareness and efficient battle with the condition. You are not alone in this fight. Stand up and face the challenge with grace and courage! Ok, or just fake it!!

I want you to think of me as your new BFF! I'll be with you, every step of the way, and together we are going to beat this!

With love and blessings,

MJ

1

The Real Deal

There is no reason you have to Think Pink. People can choose to think however they want about breast cancer.

My philosophy is to think No pink at all!

My "No-Cancer" Mantra is: Think "No Pink!" No cancer, No pink tutus, no rah-rah holding hands, no singing Kumbaya, my Lord in support groups…

Those are awesome support ideas, but if you've been in the business-world as long as I have, proving you are "the right man for the job" as many times as I have, pink is not really an appropriate touch-point for you.

Pink may even be a deterrent to you reaching out and finding the right support; thereby causing you to feel even more lonely and more alone and lost than you ever thought possible.

So who is this book for? It's not for those that want to do the all-natural, all-healing, organic food choices of curing cancer. Although some of that is in here, I think there's so much more. It's kind of a combination of materialistic with the minimalist attitude. Nah… It's definitely about materialism…with a dash of Pampering-Holistic-Healthy living.

This book is for the people that may be opposed to all that Pink, those who may be opposed to the whole "sisterhood thing." But I say to you:

You <u>can</u> choose to "all of a sudden" change your mind, change your mindset …and change your life.

You really will save your own life when you change your mind and change your mindset. Your life will be saved!

I was able to suffer through and SURVIVE Breast Cancer by pretending I never even had cancer!

Yes, you can say that "I am into denial."

I denied Breast Cancer the right to consume my life… all the while going through multiple rounds of chemotherapy, an entire year of infusions, 6 surgeries, biopsies (more surgeries actually cutting stuff out of you,) a double mastectomy, a year of painful expander fillings, and multiple reconstruction surgeries.

If I could pretend in my mind I did not have cancer after going through ALL THAT — then so can you!

Just to be clear, I am not a nurse. I am not a technical medical assistant. I may be a Certified Health Coach (CHC) today, but in no way am I making any claims about wanting to or being able to tell you the technical/medical side of the breast cancer business.

You will hear me talk about changing your life, your mind, your body, and making better choices, but this book is not for those who want a medical directory of Breast Cancer options, (although there is some of that in here.) There are plenty of other books out there for medical research.

Seriously — if you have just been diagnosed with Breast Cancer and you think you have the time and a clear-enough mind to read a bunch of books on technical medical choices for treatments… you are kidding yourself!

I am here to tell you, "as your new BFF," (best friend forever) all about the ins and outs, the feelings, the tips, and the mistakes to avoid in Breast Cancer. I will share with you what I had to go through in breast cancer and what would I recommend for you to do differently.

AS A FORMAL DISCLAIMER: EVERYTHING you read in my BFF guide to breast cancer should only be acted upon in consultation with your doctor.

Actually, I would recommend you consult with several doctors …starting first with your Breast Cancer Surgeon AND IMMEDIATELY several Breast Reconstruction Surgeons, then an Oncologist whom your doctor recommends — before you make any choices about your path to being cancer-free.

It's the final outcome that should drive your front-end research. So, start with a great reconstruction surgeon (in your health insurance network) that will advise and dictate the course of your breast surgeries. It's the "final package" that should be considered the most important .... Almost as important as the elimination of cancer in your body .... Ok ... almost.

Ah, but then I digress to the materialistic side of me…always wanting to Look Good, Feel Better! I am a walking ad for the American Cancer Society, aren't I!

Ok BFF, here is my story...

I was diagnosed with **I**nvasive **D**uctal **C**arcinoma. Nearly 80 percent of all women with breast cancer are diagnosed with **IDC**.

My tumor was "triple-negative" to hormone receptors, meaning I could not have the less invasive hormone therapy cancer treatment. (Nor can I have any hormone therapy replacement for the rest of my life for these nasty night sweats due to menopause!)

NOPE, I had to go full-blown into TCH Chemotherapy.

Because of my tumor size and the fact it had spread to outside of the breast ducts (invasive ductal,) my awesome oncologist (love her!) recommended I undergo multiple Chemotherapy treatments before my breast surgery to reduce the size of the tumor and see if the chemotherapy was being effective in killing my cancer.

That way they could see if the tumor was reducing in size. It would give a good read if the chemo was reducing the cancer and any other small cancer cells floating throughout my body. You see breast ducts drain into our lymph nodes which drain into the blood stream... Which is basically a highway for transporting cancer cells all over your body and to other organs.)

During Chemotherapy Treatments in the huge Chemo-ward in Los Angeles, I remember one of my favorite BFFs coming with me to the long drawn out 8 hour chemotherapy drug infusions. The ultimately boring, horrific experience of chemo. This is a true friend who can suffer through that with you!

Each time I underwent chemo we would immediately leave and go shopping or have a late lunch or early dinner together somewhere fabulous and very Beverly Hills-ish.

This would, of course, be based on how I was feeling after chemo. Thanks to the Zofran drug and steroids I never seemed to mind food and gained nearly 40 pounds during Chemotherapy. (There is always good news and bad news. Good that I could still feel well enough to eat…Bad that I was able to eat so much!)   I was openly hoping that Chemotherapy would finally be the means for me to lose that last 20 pounds I had been trying to shed since having two kids after forty! The great "Chemo-diet." Not!

So, shopping was a safer bet after those early on chemo sessions. Then later more sleeping consumed my life as the multiple chemotherapy treatment sessions progressed and the chemo treatments felt worse and worse. (It accumulates in your body, and feels like a terrible aching flu that comes every three weeks, with the treatments.)

I say chemo is boring because you are at the beck and call of those wonderful oncology nurses all day ... waiting for them to take your blood, waiting for them to get your pharmacy drugs ordered, waiting for them to help the other 30 patients in the "Chemo-ward," waiting for them to come in to start the IV infusion process of the chemo drugs, waiting between each bag replacement for each TCH chemo drug or saline or Benadryl bag full of IV fluids, and then more waiting for someone to turn off the annoying beeping beeping beeping of the IV pump when it gets jammed or nears the end of an IV bag. Did I mention waiting?

Let's just say there is A-LOT of waiting during Breast Cancer… waiting for this to all be over, that is!

Intra-Venus Benadryl helps with possible drug reactions ... But one great side effect is its ability to put you to sleep through the grueling 8 hours ahead of you. I loved that!

Wow, I wish there were drugs to help you go to sleep for the whole one to two YEAR process of getting through Breast Cancer Treatments and Surgeries. Then, you could just "wake up" having returned from deep space in a Sci-Fi movie on the starship enterprise, arriving at your final destination, all-perfect again with perky boobs. Dream On.

After multiple chemotherapy treatments were finished, I proceeded with an entire year of a Herceptin drug that fights fast growing cancer. Luckily Herceptin is less damaging and I felt less sick after each treatment than what I suffered through in Chemotherapy.

Because of my family history of Breast Cancer, I felt it was better for me to choose a Double Mastectomy. Even though I had interviewed two or three breast surgeons, I "only" met with one Reconstructive Surgeon who I had no idea was from "the old school" of thought on the subject.

Yes it's great that my cancer was completely removed. For that I am forever grateful. But in hindsight, I wish someone had told me that the Breast Reconstruction choices should ultimately be what <u>drives</u> your end result.

You would think that your desired end result would be killing and removing cancer from your body, right? No silly, it's Beauty! Because once the cancer is gone and they have "torn down paradise to put up a parking lot," (like the old song says,) you only have yourself to live with and you need to be happy with what you see when you look in the mirror.

I didn't know much about nipple retention and the choice of having breast implant replacement <u>at the exact same time as when you get double mastectomy surgery.</u>

Unfortunately, my Double Mastectomy was extremely invasive, with my doctor having removed way more tissue than necessary (into the clavicle and under the arms,) so I was forced to undergo an unnecessarily lengthy 12-hour reconstructive surgery following months and months of painful saline filling of expanders to stretch the muscles.

"Lucky" for me I already suffered through the year of chemo before my Double Mastectomy, so I was "fortunate" to be somewhat stronger in preparing for the horrific experience of removing my entire boobs and nipples from my body, leaving mounds of extra rolls of sagging skin while carved out tissue created baseball sized divots into my décolleté chest wall.

I was not given any alternative other than inserting expanders that are hard plastic "inflatable" reservoirs awaiting the next reconstructive surgery. It felt like each saline refill of those expanders nearly pushed and stretched my entire rib cage out to make room for silicone implants. Ouch!

Had I met my newest Reconstructive Surgeon earlier, I would have avoided these drastic painful mistakes of multiple reconstructive surgeries as a result of having just interviewed one Reconstructive Surgeon, creating the end-game and end-result first.

Love those male doctors and medical technicians in charge of saline expansion who tell you, "this won't hurt a bit, you'll feel kind of a pinch and tightness." What?! Are you kidding me?

If that were true, I guess my childbirth c-section was actually like the prick of a finger? I don't think so! No wonder they prescribe you heavy prescription muscle relaxers and Vicodin each time they inflate your "rubber tires" expanders inside you.

I am now realizing there are a lot of steps women should know that could change the way they choose their doctors and choose their treatments which would make for a much happier experience through the most fearful, painful, trying times of Breast Cancer.

Some of my choices were easy and helpful through the process, while in retrospect, I wish some of my choices had been done differently.

That is why I am here to tell you my story and help guide you like one of my closest best friends forever. And I want you to know, that for a long time I was not strong enough emotionally to share my breast cancer experiences and trials without crying a river. I wasn't strong enough to relive the experience.

2

Explaining Breast Cancer: What the ..?

While one in eight women will be diagnosed with Breast Cancer, not everyone is aware about the true identity and cause of this condition. So, to help them out with better understanding of breast cancer, let's start with a basic explanation.

What Is Breast Cancer?
Breast Cancer refers to the uncontrolled development of breast cells.

In order to better and further understand breast cancer, it may help to initially understand the process of development occurring in any cancer.

Cancer may take place due to the abnormal changes or mutations within the genes, which are responsible for cell growth regulation and maintaining their health. These genes are inside the nucleus of each cell, serving as the so called "control room" of every cell.

Basically, the cells inside your body have themselves replaced through a systematic course of cell development. In this process, healthy new cells will take over once the old ones vanish.

Over time, these abnormal changes or mutations may "turn on" particular genes, while they "turn off" others within a cell. A mutated cell sometimes obtains the capability to keep separating without order or control, creating more cells just like itself, and thus produces a tumor.

A tumor may be benign, (aka not risky) to one's health, or it may be malignant, which means it has the possibility to become dangerous.

A benign tumor is not considered cancerous, as their cells are quite close to a normal appearance. They also grow gradually and don't invade close tissues or move into to other body parts.

On the other hand, malignant tumors are known to be cancerous. Left unmonitored, malignant cells may eventually spread further than the typical tumor, sometimes to other parts of a carrier's body.

The name "breast cancer" denotes a malignant tumor which has grown from cells inside the breast.

Typically, a breast cancer can either start inside the cells of lobules, (the glands that produce milk,) or the ducts, (which are passages draining milk from the milk-producing glands to the nipple.)

Rarely, breast cancer may set off inside the stromal tissues that include the fibrous connective and fatty tissues of the breast.

In due course, cancer cells may invade healthy breast tissue close at hand and steer their way to lymph nodes of the underarm, which are small organs that have the role to filter out unknown and unneeded substances inside the body.

When cancer cells find their way into those lymph nodes, they will then get into the blood channel, accessing other body parts. The stage of the breast cancer refers to the extent of the spread of the cancer cells further than the underlying tumor.

Breast cancer has always been caused by some genetic abnormality or an error within the genetic material.

5% to 10% of cancers are because of an abnormality that is inherited from parents (mother or father). Between 85% and 90% of breast cancer conditions are because of genetic abnormalities, which occur due to the given process of aging as well as the normal "deterioration" of life as a whole.

There are a number of steps that each individual may take in order for his/her body to remain as healthy as possible. These steps include having a well balanced diet, keeping a healthy weight, limiting alcohol, regular exercising, not smoking, and more. Doing these are important. Even though they cannot get rid of the risk, they might have some effect on your possibility of acquiring breast cancer.

Did you hear that? If you can make changes to your mindset, your lifestyle, your eating, your health… You can reduce your chances of cancer!   Wow, if only I had my life to live all over again, what changes I would make!

3

Risk Factors of Developing Breast Cancer

Sometimes, developing breast cancer can be inevitable since there are certain risk factors that you might not be able to avoid. Even so, you still need to be aware about the different risk factors of having breast cancer. This will allow you to avoid, if possible, and identify some of the preventive measures in order to at least make the condition better.

Identifying Your Risk Factors

Different cancers have different risk factors.

For instance, having your skin exposed to too much sunlight can be a risk factor for developing skin cancer. Frequent smoking can be a risk factor for cancer of the mouth, voice box, larynx, lung, kidney, bladder, and a number of other organs.

However, risk factors might not tell you everything. Having risk factors does not necessarily mean that you will acquire a disease.

A majority of women having one breast cancer risk factor or more never develop the condition, whereas many women suffering from the condition have no visible risk factors, apart from growing older and being a woman.

Even if a woman displaying the risk factors develops the cancer, it will still be difficult to determine just how much those factors may have contributed.

Some factors trigger possibility more than others. Furthermore, your possibility for developing breast cancer might change over time because of certain factors like lifestyle or aging.

Unchangeable Risk Factors

➤ Gender – Being a female is simply the major risk factor you may have for breast cancer development. Men can also develop the condition. However, the disease is around a hundred times more frequent among women as compared to men. Probably, this is because males have lesser of female hormones, such as progesterone and estrogen, which might promote growth for breast cancer cells.

➤ Aging – As you grow older, your possibility to develop breast cancer improves. Around 1 out of 8 persistent breast cancers are being diagnosed in women below 45, whereas 2 out of 3 persistent breast cancers are diagnosed among women aging 55 and above.

(Did you know that women with large mid-sections, (apple and pear shape) tend to rank high on risk of Breast Cancer. One more reason to 'get moving!")

➤ Genetic – Estimated 5 percent to 10 percent of total breast cancer cases are believed to be genetic or hereditary. This means that the development of the diseases has directly resulted from abnormal gene changes, known as mutations, inherited from one's parent.

Angelina Jolie has recently made public her testing positive for the BRCA1 gene, which increased her chance of having Breast Cancer by nearly 85% risk .

➤ Breast Cancer Family History – The possibility of developing breast cancer is greater among women who have close blood relatives having the disease. Having a first-degree relative (daughter, sister, or mother) who suffers from breast cancer roughly doubles the risk of a woman. Having two first-degree relatives elevate her risk around 3-fold.

After my Breast Cancer biopsy came back positive for Invasive Ductal Carcinoma, I learned from my family that my Grandmother and Great Aunt on my father's side had both been diagnosed with breast cancer. Ask about your family history.

➤ Breast Cancer Personal History – A patient who has cancer in a breast has around 3-4 times higher risk for developing cancer in her other breast or within another section of similar breast. The condition may be different from a return or recurrence of a first cancer.

This is why I chose to have a double mastectomy," Who in their right mind would want to go through the nightmare twice?!?"

➤ Ethnicity And Race – In general, white women are determined to be more likely to acquire breast cancer as compared with African-American women. On the other hand, African-American women diagnosed with Breast Cancer were reported to have higher death rates due to breast cancer. Amongst women who are 45 years old or below, breast cancer is more likely to develop among African-American women. Hispanic, Native American, and Asian women hold a lower possibility of dying from breast cancer.

Aside from these, there are many risk factors of breast cancer that are unchangeable or unavoidable. Now, let's see what risk factors you can change…

Lifestyle-Related Breast Cancer Risk Factors

➤ Birth Control – Using oral contraceptives can increase your breast cancer risk factor. In fact, women who use them hold some greater risk on developing the disease as compared with women who don't use them.

(Yep, I took The Pill for years!)

➤ Having Kids - Women who have had no children or the ones who get their first one after the age of 30 have a bit higher risk for developing breast cancer. Having a number of pregnancies and being pregnant at young age decrease the possibility of having breast cancer. Pregnancy decreases the total number of a woman's lifetime menstrual cycles that might be the root for such effect.

Yes, I had both my kids near the age of 40, not to mention I also took all the drugs at an earlier age for reproductive In-Vitro Fertilization. Yikes …we haven't even touched the surface about the IVF hormone havoc contributions to Breast Cancer.

➢ Breastfeeding – A few studies have suggested that breastfeeding might slightly decrease the risk of breast cancer, particularly when it has been continued for 1½ up to 2 years. A certain explanation for such potential effect might include the fact that breastfeeding lessens the total number of a woman's lifetime menstrual cycles, as does having kids.

Yes again, I was a pitiful breast-feeding mother who suffered from breast mastitis and quit in the first few months following childbirth.

➢ Drinking Alcohol – The consumption of alcohol is apparently related to increased possibility of breast cancer development. This possibility increases through the amount of consumed alcohol. As compared with nondrinkers, women who consume a single alcoholic drink each day have an extremely slight increase in possibility. However, too much alcohol consumption is also determined to boost the possibility of developing many other forms of cancer.

Guilty here!

➢ Overweight -- The Old Spare — a large mid-section of the woman's body increases risk of Breast Cancer.

Along with these, certain physical activities, obesity or being overweight (Guilty!), and many others may also contribute to the increasing or decreasing the risk of breast cancer development.

So, get to know these and understand them better, as they can help you discover more about the occurrence of Breast Cancer and how to avoid being in the high risk group.

Now it's all coming together... So far I am 0 for 5, no wonder I had Breast Cancer.

4

Food & Exercise Issues Related to Breast Cancer

Just like other kinds of health conditions, breast cancer requires the right type of food and exercise in order to be prevented, and can be encouraged by "poor" choices of food and exercise routine.

The choices you made about what you did or didn't do with your body very likely had something to do with you experiencing this disease.

Eat Right and Move Right Moving Forward

Once you have been diagnosed with breast cancer, it can greatly affect your emotional and physical health. Maintaining a healthy lifestyle is truly important.

By eating the right foods containing high amounts of anti-oxidants and exercising regularly, you are on your way to helping your body heal and saving your precious vessel from having to deal with more dangerous toxins.

The following can be your guideline to taking the right path:

Exercise

An analysis combining the results of 31 studies on physical activity and breast cancer found that the women who did the most activity had a 12% lower risk of developing breast cancer compared with the least active women. The analysis also showed that the more activity a woman does, the more she can reduce her risk of breast cancer. For example, for every 2 hours a week a woman spends doing moderate to vigorous activity, the risk of breast cancer falls by 5%.

➤ Walking – According to professionals, walking 2 to 3 miles every day can reduce your risk of breast cancer by as much as 40%. This activity may also help you fight depression, fatigue, and anxiety. It can also help you improve bone and heart health.

➤ Pilates – Some people believe that Pilates could even aid with concentration, centering, flow, breath and control that give connections between your mind and body.

➤ Yoga – Based on a study, a number of breast cancer survivors who have attended 2 yoga classes each week for three months after their treatment felt less fatigued and held lesser inflammation as compared to women who didn't attend the class. Performing yoga activities may help ease depression, fatigue and pain among women who are fighting against breast cancer. It also serves as a great source of relaxation and meditation. (we all know that stress is one of the major contributing factors to Breast Cancer.)

➤ Meditation – exercise your brain, focus on peace, clearing your mind, and reducing the stress in your life. (we all know that stress is one of the leading causes of Breast Cancer.) Think "No Pink."

Food

The old adage "We are what we eat" has never been more true than it is today, when scientists are continuously alerting us about the link between diet and disease.

Whether you are trying to overcome cancer or trying to avoid it, there are a multitude of dietary suggestions to give you a fighting edge against this life-threatening disease. In this section, we'll cover a list of foods and dietary habits that are conducive to supporting your fight against cancer.

More than just a listing of foods you should eat or should avoid, scientists and researchers come to an agreement on a listing of nutrients which are imperative for fighting cancer. Regardless of where or how you consume these nutrients, they should become a vital part of your dietary intake.

Essential Cancer-Fighting Nutrients:

- ➤ Folate-Rich Foods: Folate is part of the Vitamin B Complex and is believed to ward off some cancer-inducing DNA mutations. Many manufacturers of cereals, breads and pastas fortify their foods with this nutrient and it is naturally found in orange juice, leafy green vegetables and dried beans.

- ➤ Vitamin D: This fat-soluble vitamin is thought to curb the growth of cancerous cells. Often associated with milk, equally high concentrations of vitamin D can be found seafood (e.g. cod, shrimp and salmon) and by soaking in natural sunlight through the skin.

Food Choices with Cancer-Fighting Properties:

➤ Tea: Tea contains flavonoids which are known for their antioxidant effect. Antioxidants are thought to tie up free radicals released through routine cellular metabolism which, left in a free state, can cause damage to DNA. A diet rich in antioxidants, of which tea is an example, is thought to be protective and defensive against cancer. Hot and cold, black and green varieties of tea are all thought to contain fairly equal amounts of antioxidants.

➤ Cruciferous Vegetables: There may have been something to your mom telling you to "eat your broccoli!" Broccoli, kale, turnip greens, cabbage, cauliflower and Brussels sprouts, are all part of a group of vegetables known as cruciferous vegetables, which are all part of the cabbage family.

In research studies, a substance found in these vegetables has suggested they produce cancer-killing effects, especially in prostate and colon cancer varieties.

Interestingly, swallowing these vegetables whole does not release the ingredient with cancer-fighting properties and one must actually chew or at least dice the vegetable to realize its cancer-fighting benefits.

➤ Curcumin: This bright, yellow spice is probably one you've had before and perhaps didn't know it. A main ingredient in curry powder, curcumin is a common addition to rice, chicken, vegetables, lentils and Indian foods.

A common cancer denominator in most patients is the presence of chronic tissue inflammation. Curcumin is believed to have anti-inflammatory effects, thereby greatly reducing the risk of developing cancer. For those fighting cancer, it also has benefit in that it is thought to interfere with cell-signaling pathways, suppressing the transformation, proliferation and invasion of cancerous cells.

➤ Ginger: Both grated and whole ginger root have showed promise as a cancer-fighting food. Many are familiar with ginger as it relates to aiding digestion. Interestingly, this is precisely the same effect it has on cancer cells in some research studies: ginger actually tricks the cancer cells into digesting themselves without harming the surrounding, normal cells of the body. Ginger makes a nice addition to marinades, soups and smoothies, and it's also widely available as a tea and as a gingered ale beverage.

➤ Garlic: There have been several large studies concluding that those who eat garlic daily are less likely to develop cancer and that those who are fighting cancer have had benefit in minimizing cancer cell growth by eating garlic. There isn't consensus on how much garlic to eat daily, but researchers do agree that it's the garlic clove that should be consumed, not garlic salt or garlic powder, to achieve maximum results.

➤ Berries: High in cancer-fighting antioxidants, berries also contain compounds which help keep cancers from growing or spreading. Berries are readily available year-round in most grocery stores; if not available fresh, try an organic, frozen option instead. Add them to smoothies or to cereal or yogurt for a treat, or eat them whole. All varieties of berries are considered helpful in an anti-cancer diet.

➤ Grapes: Within the skin of red grapes is a rich source of the antioxidant resveratrol. Found also in grape juice and red wine, resveratrol is thought to be helpful in keeping cancer away and keeping cancer from spreading. In men especially, moderate consumption of red wine is thought to be preventative for prostate cancer.

➤ Beans: Because of their rich source of antioxidants and folate, beans are not only a smart choice for a high-fiber, low-fat diet, they are also recommended as part of an anti-cancer diet. Organic and non-GMO varieties are available and they are a highly versatile food to incorporate into your diet.

<u>A few Foods to Start Getting You on the Right Track:</u>

➤ Whole Grains – This type of food is believed to help people with breast cancer. You can go for whole grains like barley, quinoa, brown rice, amaranth, whole wheat, and oats, which contain more minerals, vitamins, and fiber.

➤ Tomatoes – According to some studies, consuming fresh tomatoes can safeguard post-menstrual women against breast cancer. Researchers have determined that eating lots of tomatoes can produce some increase in the formation of hormones, which control the fat and sugar metabolism of your body.

Other foods that have been determined to aid in improving your overall wellbeing and health include:

➤ Berries – Berries have antioxidants that decrease the formation of cancer cells inside the body. Raspberries, strawberries, or blueberries are great choices for snacks or something you would want to add into your regular meals.

➤ Coconut Oil, Cinnamon, Tumeric

➤ Salmon – Fresh Wild Salmon has great content of Omega-3s, and Vitamin D and B12. It can offer you body with the right nutrients it requires for regulating cell development and aid as part of your breast cancer prevention diet.

<u>Cancer-Causing Foods to Avoid</u>:

There is a hefty list of foods one should definitely avoid in the fight against cancer. Many of these are every day foods that are suspected of causing cancer directly or contain carcinogens that can lead to development of cancer.

> Microwave Popcorn: It's so convenient to pop a bag of popcorn in the microwave, isn't it? But did you know that microwave popcorn is a danger to your health in several ways?

The bag is lined with a chemical called perfluorooctanoic acid (PFOA), a chemical also found in Teflon, which is known to cause cancer in lab animals when heated. The EPA has listed this chemical as a known carcinogen.

Unless labeled otherwise, the popcorn itself most likely uses soybean oil and a preservative of propyl gallate, both of which have been linked to cancer.

> Non-Organic Fruits: Fruits not labeled as Organic are contaminated with pesticides such as atrazine, thiodicarb and organophosphates. These chemicals have been demonstrated to not only cause cancer but also diminish the reproductive capabilities of humans. Unfortunately, washing fruits prior to eating them doesn't remove all of the chemical and the only way to avoid these toxic and carcinogenic substances is to buy Certified Organic fruits.

➤ Canned Tomatoes: Avoid canned tomatoes at all costs! The lining of the can contains bisphenol-A (BPA) which is leeched from the lining into the tomatoes themselves by the exceptionally high acidity inherent to tomatoes. BPA has been demonstrated to affect the way genes work in the brain of rats, leaving them more susceptible to cancer.

➤ Processed Meats: This category encompasses a wide range of meats common in most grocery stores, including sausages, hot dogs, bacon, lunch meats, bologna and pimento loaves. It is commonly believed that the chemicals and preservatives (e.g., sodium nitrates are quite common) act as carcinogens. Sodium nitrate-free meats can be found, but not as easily. They have a shorter shelf-like but are devoid of the cancer-causing effects of their processed counterparts.

➤ Farmed Salmon: Once thought to be one of the healthiest foods on the planet, salmon has a deadly secret: when farmed, as opposed to caught in the wild, salmon is contaminated with chemicals, antibiotics and pesticides, as well as carcinogens. Studies have indicated that farmed salmon contains high levels of cancer-causing dioxins which can be avoided by buying wild caught salmon instead.

➤ Potato Chips: This quick, crispy snack is one we know to avoid due to its high content of fat and calories. But did you know that the process of frying potatoes at high temperatures to make them crispy also causes them to make a substance called acrylamide? Acrylamide is a known carcinogen also found in cigarettes. Try air-popped popcorn or whole wheat pretzels as an alternative to these carcinogenic crunchy treats.

➤ Hydrogenated Oils: Drop the long name and what you really have here is vegetable oil. Unlike butter, vegetable oils must undergo a chemical process in order extract their fats into a usable form that giant corporations are able to then package and sell to you, the unsuspecting public. The process of extracting this oil, also known as hydrogenation, is thought to influence our cells' membrane structure, an occurrence which has been linked to cancer.

➤ Highly salted, pickled or smoked foods: This category encompasses bacon, sausage, bologna and salami as well as pickled foods and smoked nuts. Curing food in this fashion causes us to intake N-nitrosol composites which have been associated with an increased risk of developing cancers.

➤ Highly Processed White Flour: Many people have adopted a diet lower in processed white flour simply as a means of encouraging themselves to eat more whole grains. And that's a good thing! The glycemic index of processed flour is very high, meaning consuming it raises insulin levels quickly and encourages high blood sugar. Since cancerous tumors feed mostly on sugars in the bloodstream, limiting blood sugar levels is a great way to starve tumors and discourage their growth.

➤ Genetically Modified Organisms (GMOs): Many foods available to us now have been modified by chemicals and grown with chemicals, especially most grains (e.g., soybeans, wheat, corn). And, these grains are fed to factory-farmed animals, so they show up in our meat as well.

Most of the rest of the world has banned the use of GMOs in their food stream, but so far the United States has not. In lab studies, rats fed GMO foods showed damaged immune systems, precancerous cell growth and smaller brains and livers in just 10 days, 100% of the time.

GMOs are a huge concern among many consumers trying to retain good health, avoid cancer and treat cancer. Unfortunately, there is no requirement to label foods as containing GMOs, so it's difficult to find foods that don't unless they specifically state "GMO free" or "no GMO."

➤ Refined Sugar: Similar to the argument made against refined white flour, refined sugar is also a no-no for those battling cancer or trying to avoid it. The spike in blood sugar levels as a result of consuming refined sugar provides a feeding ground for tumor cells. High-fructose corn syrup is particularly harmful as it is the "food of choice" for cancer cells in that it is metabolized quickly and easily.

➤ Artificial Sweeteners: Anything you use to achieve a sweet taste in your food or beverage besides refined sugar is probably artificial (except honey, molasses or maple syrup). Aspartame is chief among this group (think Diet Coke, Diet Pepsi, most diet sodas). Aspartame and other chemical sweeteners are thought break down in the body into DKP, a deadly toxin that has been linked to cancer and especially brain tumors.

➤ Alcohol: Limited alcohol consumption, especially wine, is thought to be useful in maintaining good health. Anything beyond moderate or low consumption however has been linked as a main cause of a variety of cancers, including mouth, esophagus, liver, colon, rectal and breast cancer.

Excessive alcohol use is considered the second leading cause of cancer, second only to tobacco use.

➤ Red Meat: Prolonged and regular consumption of red meat has been linked to increased risk of colon cancer, whereas choosing a lighter animal protein (e.g. poultry, fish) has been shown to be protective against cancer. When you do occasionally enjoy a good cut of red meat, be sure that it is from a grass fed source to avoid byproducts of GMO grain consumption in your meat.

➤ Soda: Beyond having a load of sugar or artificial sweetener in it, soda has its own reason for being on the "avoid" list. Many sodas contain artificial colorings and food chemicals (e.g., derivative 4-methylimidazole or 4-MI) which have been linked to esophageal and stomach cancers as well.

If you consume any of these (as I did, and regretfully still do), please know you truly will become one of the "High-risk women" — with possibly unusual results — who might require additional tests or need frequent and earlier screening for Breast Cancer.

With such long lists of things to eat or avoid, it can be difficult to create an eating plan that is balanced, affordable and cancer-fighting all rolled into one.

Truly, there seems to be a lot to think about when it comes to knowing how to choose your foods while balancing your pocket book, your health and your time.

It's advisable not to try and tackle the entire list of Do's and Don'ts all at once. Instead, choose one item off this list to incorporate into your lifestyle each week and gradually, over time, you will find what works for you, what you can afford, and what is of the utmost importance to you individually in your cancer battle plan.

But do something with this list; don't disregard the wisdom researchers have gained in linking diet to cancer.

Truly, we are what we eat and diet is becoming unarguably one of the largest risks for developing cancer of any of our lifestyle choices.

Make your own list of Foods you would like to take out of your diet and replace with new "CANCER FREE Foods"

_____
_____
_____
_____
_____
_____
_____
_____
_____
_____
_____
_____
_____
_____
_____
_____
_____
_____
_____
_____
_____
_____
_____
_____
_____
_____
_____
_____

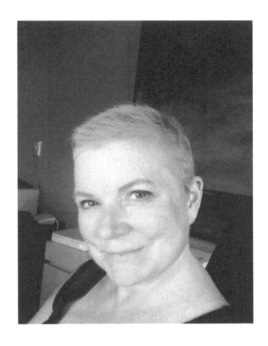

Just like waiting for your hair to grow back after Chemotherapy, Patience is a virtue! Making life saving changes to your diet should be taken one step at a time. Small improvements taken each day and even a week at a time could save your life and need to be permanent LIFESTYLE changes for the rest of your AMAZING life!

Chapter 5

Breast Cancer Diagnosis and Tests

Early detection of the disease could be a huge plus in fighting breast cancer. It's essential that you know about the different breast cancer tests and diagnoses for better chances of survival.

Early Diagnosis of Breast Cancer

The earlier breast cancer is identified, the better it can be for the long-term health of the patient. For women, who are at average risk of breast cancer, clinical exams, mammography, and self-exams starting at 30 years old, can screen for the disease. High-risk women or unusual results might require additional tests or earlier screening.

Tests

> Breast Self-Exam – Doing regular breast self-examinations is a practical and essential grass-roots way to aid in taking care of yourself, and it's vitally important that you regularly examine your breast personally to know if there are changes to the shape or size of your breast. Usually, you are the one who will know first if there is something wrong with your breast.

It is highly recommended that women do breast self-examination at least once a month. The recommended time to conduct breast self-examination is one week after the start of your monthly period.

There are two ways that you can use when conducting breast self-examination: sight and touch.

You need to look at and feel your breast to know if there are some changes that took place in your breast. There are two things that you should remember when conducting breast self-examination:

1. LOOK: When conducting breast self-examination it is essential that you use a mirror so that you check your breast. Check if there are lumps, pulls, and skin color changes to your breast. Leaning forward and standing upright is the best position to conduct breast self-examination. You need to remember that your breasts must look the same particularly around the area of your nipples.

2. FEEL: When conducting breast self-examination, it is also essential that you feel your breast. There are two parts when conducting this step. The first method is the use of oil or water on your breast area. Oil or water can help you so that your finger can slide easily around the area of your breast. You can do breast self examination while taking a bath or while you are in the shower. Move your fingers around each breast in a clockwise and counter-clockwise motion. Feeling every inch of breast tissue and seeing if there are any hard spots or lumps.

- ➤ Mammogram – This test is a specialized form of X-ray performed to find unusual changes or growths within breast tissue. It can be the main tool in detecting breast cancer, although no particular test is flawless.

- ➤ Clinical Breast Exam – This form of breast exam is conducted by a medical professional. It is an underlying part of the checkups of women, starting at the age of 20.

- ➤ Breast Ultrasound – Sometimes, medical professionals utilize ultrasound images for checking if a certain breast lump is a cyst or a hard mass.

- ➤ Breast MRI – Stands for Magnetic Resonance Imaging and is used as an aid for detecting breast cancer.

- ➤ Minimally Invasive Breast Biopsy – This form of breast biopsy normally applies a needle and not surgery.

- ➤ Breast Biopsy – When professionals conduct a biopsy, they eliminate cells from the suspicious mass to determine if it is cancer.

- ➤ Ductal Lavage – This procedure includes monitoring of cells from milk ducts for precancerous cells.

- ➤ Sentinel Node Biopsy – Within a sentinel node biopsy, medical professionals check some lymph nodes beneath the arm to identify if cancer has already spread in the lymph system.

These are only some of the many breast cancer diagnosis and tests you can find around. Please check with your Doctor and learn more about which ones best suits your needs.

In my case, I had dense breasts with silicone implants. My mammogram did not detect the mass of cancer. It wasn't until I had a "sugar seeking infusion MRI" that I became aware of the killer cells living and growing inside my body.

The technician could see the sugar induced fluid being sucked into the black vacant looking mass on the screen. Cancer feeds on sugar!

With that black blob identified, it was then important for me to do an ultrasound to measure the size of the mass in question.

Next came a biopsy of the area.

Remember: "High-risk women or unusual results might require additional tests or earlier screening."

If you consume any of the high risk Lifestyle choices of Cancer-Causing Foods or have a history of Unchangeable Risk Factors such as age, family history, BRCA genes, or you hold any one of the Lifestyle-Related Breast Cancer Risk Factors such as having used birth control or frequently drinking more than moderate amounts of alcohol or if you are overweight please know that you must heed my advice and seek aggressive Breast Cancer screenings earlier and often!

Chapter 6

Misconceptions About Breast Cancer

Knowing only some facts about breast cancer is a way for you to determine and apply the best ways to prevent or fight it off.

Sometimes, breast cancer misconceptions lead a lot of people to wrong decisions. This is something you don't want to happen to you, so make sure to be aware of the misconceptions in this chapter.

Misconception can Result in Taking Wrong Action

For sure, there is increased knowledge and increased awareness about breast cancer today. There is still, however, misinformation and confusion around the issue.

The following are some of the common misconceptions about breast cancer:

➤ Breast Pain Is A Breast Cancer Symptom. This is hardly ever the case. Particularly, early stage breast cancer normally does not cause pain and might display no evident symptoms. Most pains, tenderness or aches may be attributed to circumstances like fibrocystic breast development and the swell of hormones, among other causes.

➤ You Are Merely At Risk When Breast Cancer Runs Within Your Family. Only 5% to 10% of total breast cancer cases are hereditary because of mutations within genes linked with the condition.

➤ Regular Self-Exams Don't Make Any Difference. Performing regular breast checkups should be an essential part of every woman's anti-cancer precautions and prevention plans.

➤ Breast Cancer Is Only Possible Among Women. Even though women account for the huge majority of breast cancer cases, men can also be susceptible. Most famously, the character Dr. Christian Troy on the hit TV series Nip/Tuck suffered from breast cancer on the show.

➤ Underwire, Tight Bras Result In Breast Cancer. This misconception started with the idea claiming that wearing tight fitting bras all day long on a daily basis can contribute to lymphatic drainage issues in women, hence, trapping toxins within the breast tissue. However, scientists have discounted the theory through its failure to leave out confounding variables, including the presence in some females with determined risk factors for breast cancer.

➤ Women With Fibrocystic, Lumpy Breasts Have Higher Risk. In the past, this has been considered to increase your risk, but not today. However, lumpy breasts do make it harder to distinguish typical tissues from the cancerous ones. Therefore, it is still a good move to talk to a medical professional about this concern.

Make sure that the things you believe about breast cancer are fact and not just misconceptions in order for it to lead you to a better health status, toward the highest level of wellness and away from the risk of breast cancer.

Chapter 7

Medical Professional Breast Cancer Consultation

Getting a medical professional breast cancer consultation is essential in order to increase your chances of surviving breast cancer. There are several medical breast cancer centers that you can rely on in terms of getting the best breast cancer treatment.

To ensure that you can acquire the best breast cancer diagnosis and treatment, it is essential that you get suitable and reliable medical opinion through medical professional breast cancer consultation.

If you notice breast cancer symptoms, it is highly recommended that you get the best breast cancer screening and consultation from a reliable medical expert who specializes in conducting breast examination.

There are several medical experts who specialize in breast cancer cases. Most of them believe that proper medical breast cancer consultation is very important in order to increase the patient's chance to survive breast cancer.

Proper and accurate breast cancer consultation can save thousands of women's lives. Early detection can definitely help you minimize your risks. It is the main reason why women should take this as an advantage. Women must get proper medical breast care consultation in order to get suitable breast cancer diagnosis and treatment.

I suggest you only work with medical professionals who specialize in breast cancer cases.

When to Get Breast Cancer Consultation?

Breast cancer symptoms may vary person to person. Lump(s) in the breast, fluid in the nipple(s), changes in the shape of your breast, discolored patches in the breast area and dimpling of your skin in the breast area are common symptoms of breast cancer.

The last stage of breast cancer manifests yellow skin, the occurrence of lymph nodes, and pain in the bone. But such symptoms usually occur during the second or last stage of breast cancer, and this is the main reason why most women with breast cancer are being diagnosed during the last stage of the disease.

Diagnosing breast cancer during its last stage can lower the patient's chance of survival. That's how important early breast cancer detection is.

Chapter 8

Possible Treatments & Surgeries

So, you are diagnosed with breast cancer. What will you do now?

To be diagnosed with breast cancer is indeed a tough situation that not all women can endure. It is not easy to have breast cancer because you need to go through physical, emotional and even mental changes.

It is normal to feel scared or in denial once you know that you have it. You will feel scared because you do not want to die and leave your loved ones.

For sure, you will feel sacred about the possible pain that you might experience when your disease progresses.

Probably, you will experience a denial stage. (I did very well for myself by staying in denial almost the entire time! LOL)

To be sure, you may consider getting a second, third, or fourth opinion from other doctors. I highly recommend this. It is a smart choice to get multiple opinions and diagnosis so that you know whether your first diagnosis is accurate or not.

There are some cases where opinion and diagnosis of doctors are inaccurate. You should get multiple opinions so that you can get accurate and reliable medical advice and have a clear understanding <u>for yourself</u> of which path to take.

Now is the time to start accepting that you have breast cancer and be ready to face it.

Your life does not end the moment that you get diagnosed with breast cancer. You are still breathing and there is still a hope for a complete cure (technically they call it remission... but I am of the firm belief that if you have early stage Breast Cancer, get a double mastectomy along with a year of chemotherapy and herceptin treatments, your chances are higher that you will be cured. Please consult with your doctor.)

Strong family support is very important so that a person with breast cancer can get a sense of motivation, love, and inspiration to continue fighting against breast cancer.

Aside from family support, the desire of a person to live can also help her acquire strength to survive. Women diagnosed with breast cancer should get breast cancer treatments and surgeries in order to acquire total recovery from this disease.

Breast Cancer Treatments

Through medical advancement and modernization, there are now several breast cancer treatments and surgeries for patients who are diagnosed with breast cancer. You need to know that breast cancer treatments may vary in accordance to the size and type of tumor in your breast.

Medical experts who specialize in handling breast cancer cases will know the best type(s) of treatment for your case.

Please note (as mentioned previously,) it is critical to interview several doctors to gain your own opinion of the path you would like to take for Breast Cancer Treatment. Start with the Breast Reconstructive Surgeon to begin the formation of your medical team, and you will be much happier in the end.

The Reconstructive Surgeon usually drives the type of final outcome you are looking for. Please start there and ask whether to have nipple retention, whether you are a candidate for one stop surgery, (a mastectomy and reconstructive surgery all at the same time,) or do they recommend for you to have two surgeries with the insertion of breast expanders at time of double mastectomy (old school.)

Medical experts will consider the size of the tumor, type of cancer, any affected lymph nodes via a PET Scan, and other important factors relevant to your disease. Other health issues, personal preferences, family history, Hormone therapy, your age, and the status of your menstrual periods are also important factors that your doctor will consider so that he or she can give the best breast cancer treatment that suits your case and condition.

Breast cancer treatments have two major goals; to eliminate the cancer cells inside your body, and to prevent its recurrence.

There are several breast cancer treatments that may suit your case.

Types of Breast Cancer Treatment

1. Surgery – Can be either lumpectomy or mastectomy. There are also several types of lumpectomies and mastectomies.

2. Chemotherapy - Chemotherapy is a type of therapy that also uses drugs that can kill the cancer cells. Patients who get this type of therapy may experience some side effects such as fatigue, hot flashes, hair loss, nausea and many more.

3. Biological therapy - Works by improving the patient's immune system. It can also kill the cancer cells.

4. Hormone therapy - Also called Endocrine therapy. It involves the use of drugs and steroids to eliminate cancer cells. This treatment comes with side effects such as vaginal dryness and hot flashes.

5. Radiation therapy - A systematic type of breast cancer treatment. It is used to lessen and eventually, destroy the cancer cells inside the patient's body.

Types of Breast Cancer Surgery

Surgeries to remove cancer may vary due to different factors.

Surgical procedures for breast cancer are:

- Modified Radical Mastectomy

- Simple Mastectomy

- Total Mastectomy

- Segmental Mastectomy

- Partial mastectomy

- Lumpectomy

Things to Consider when Getting Breast Cancer Surgeries

- You need to know that women who choose to undergo a Lumpectomy for their breast cancer usually get multiple radiation procedures in addition to chemotherapy.

- Women with early stage of Breast Cancer who choose to have a double mastectomy usually have a good chance of not needing radiation treatments.

- Women diagnosed with a large tumor may want to consider a Double Mastectomy vs. only a Lumpectomy.

- You should definitely get breast cancer reconstruction surgery at the same time or after your breast cancer surgery. It should help make you feel good again about your physical appearance after losing one or both of your breasts. And we all know, when you Look Good, you Feel Better.

Chapter 9

Tips on How to Survive Breast Cancer

To have breast cancer is a challenge that can make you feel scared and frustrated. However, due to the power of modernization and medical advancement, breast cancer patients still have fantastic rates of survival. There are many women who fought and have survived breast cancer. So, if they made it, there is a chance that you can survive too.

Here are some ways that can help you increase your chance to beat breast cancer:

- It is important that you choose the best breast cancer surgery and treatment to eliminate the cancerous cells inside your body. The suitability of the surgery and treatment that you can get may vary depending on the stage of your disease.

- Once diagnosed with Breast Cancer, choose the best medical expert team starting first with your Breast Reconstructive Surgeon before you choose what type of surgery to have. Interview several doctors who can give the best and suitable breast cancer treatment and surgery for you.

- The support of your family also plays a vital role as it motivates patients to be strong, fight and survive. The eagerness of a person to survive the disease can also contribute a lot in terms of breast cancer survival.

-    In order to survive breast cancer, it is important that you hold onto and keep your faith that you can survive. You must believe that breast cancer is just a challenge that you will overcome.

To survive a deadly disease like breast cancer is indeed a great achievement that you can and will achieve. Multiple-year cancer-free Breast Cancer survivors serve as an inspiration for all other breast cancer patients to prove they can also survive.

Chapter 10

Preventing Breast Cancer Recurrence

Breast cancer survivors must take the time to consider ways to avoid the recurrence of breast cancer.

There are several ways that can help you reduce your chances of having to deal with this nightmare again.

Here are some tips on how you can avoid breast cancer recurrence:

- Eat nutritious foods

- Get enough sleep

- Exercise

- Get regular breast cancer screenings, like a mammogram.

- Early Detection: One of the most effective ways to detect symptoms of breast cancer is through conducting breast-self examination. Women must be aware of breast cancer prevention because prevention is "way" better than treatment.

Breast cancer is potentially a death sentence. It stops you from enjoying your life and time with your loved ones.

Through breast cancer screenings, you will know the current status of your body. Changing your mindset and making better lifestyle choices will ultimately save your life by reducing your risk of breast cancer.

I now realize there are many steps women should know that could change the way they choose their doctors and choose their treatments in order to have a happier experience through the most fearful, painful, trying times of Breast Cancer. Some of my choices were easy and helpful. Some were downright genius. Others, in hindsight, were mistakes.

That is why I wanted to share my story with you and help guide you like one of my closest BFFs. Until now, I never was strong enough to share my breast cancer experiences and trials without crying a river. To my sister and to my family, I want to deeply apologize for the agony and selfishness I put you through by shutting myself out from even discussing the topic of Breast Cancer with you. I wasn't strong enough to relive the experience. I can say now, that by my choosing to think "No Pink," I not only survived, I was able to thrive!

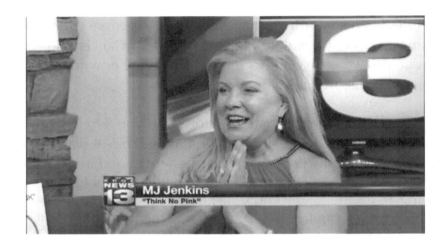

ABOUT THE AUTHOR

MJ Jenkins is a breast cancer survivor, a representative of the American Cancer Society, and a coach for women going through breast cancer. Get more information on her products and services at www.ThinkNoPink.com